How I Achieved

FREEDOM FROM ARTHRITIS

Learn the secrets that can reduce pain and increase movement in Osteoarthritis.

Eugene Sims

First published by Sims Press 2013

www.freedomfromarthritis.com

ISBN 978-15306592-10

Disclaimer

Please note this book is not a diagnostic tool. It is a guide only. It is not intended to replace qualified medical advice. Before beginning any of these suggestions you should first seek qualified medical advice.

Although muscle-based problems are easy to diagnose, a separate complication exists. That is the fact that although there may be positive muscle problems found there can also be other underlying problems. It is essential that other problems are identified so that safe and effective treatment can follow.

The author accepts no responsibility for the outcomes as a result of following the information in this book.

The names and any identifying features relating to case studies in this book are fictitious, to protect the identity of the people concerned.

Dedicated to:

My family, who have been the inspiration behind this book.

Table of Contents

Preface

It took me seven years to find something to give me relief with osteoarthritis in my knees. It took me another fifteen years before I realised that what I learned was not common knowledge – in fact it was quite uncommon.

Over time I saw that working with people one on one was a very limited way of spreading the message. Finally, in sheer frustration, I knew that I had to put this information out into the wide world, so it could benefit the millions of people who suffer from osteoarthritis.

This book aims to provide some unique and useful strategies to improve movement and reduce the pain of osteoarthritis. My hope is that it will benefit many by supplying some tangible relief from their condition.

Acknowledgements

I am blessed to have many great mentors, without whom this book may never have been finished. They include friends and family, and past mentors such as employers, lecturers and teachers.

There are too many to list without this being a book of acknowledgements. I trust that all those who have influenced me take this word of gratitude from me with love and sincere thanks.

I will make specific reference to the nearest and dearest as follows.

The encouragement and understanding of my wife is the most immediate, as well as the inspiration from my children.

For my parents who encouraged and supported me to always follow my dreams, and a big brother who gave me the inspiration to keep 'stepping up'.

Professionally I acknowledge Dr Janet G Travell, Louis S Simons and Dr David G Simons, whose work was my first glimpse into a whole new understanding of the muscles influence on our body. In this light I also thank Simon Louden, who first introduced me to this information.

Of course no written work would be possible

without a good editor: to this end I thank Gillian Tewsley. Further thanks to Gilly Clark for her expertise in proof reading. My thanks also to Glenys Bean for helpful advice and guidance; and to Joel Bauer for his expertise, which made it possible to reach the world with this information.

Last but not least, to some life may appear to be a series of 'coincidences'. I however don't believe that things happen by chance. I give thanks to my creator who, I believe, has guided me through it all.

1

My story

How it all began

I vividly remember the first time the pain struck me. I was hiking out towards the majestic Cape Brett in the Bay of Islands during the summer of 1992. It was a sharp, knife-like piercing pain behind my left kneecap. It began while I was descending a hill, as I took my weight on my left leg. I was unaware of what the pain was about – and I certainly had no idea of the journey it would lead me on, or how it would change life as I knew it.

Over the next few months the pain got worse and more frequent. I had to give up running and any sports that involved running, because the pain was so severe during the activity and for days after. Even walking up and down stairs was painful. Squatting was very painful and restricted: I could perform only half a squat, as agony prevented me from going any further.

The pain I experienced was actually two types of pain. One was a dull ache deep in the knee joint, which could be there both during movement and at rest. The other pain was the classic pain of osteoarthritis: it felt like pieces of broken glass rubbing underneath my kneecap as I walked or tried to squat.

The physical effects of the pain and its limitations also took their toll emotionally. Until this point in my life I had always been physically very active. I had been a distance runner for the previous eight years, and had loved playing all sports. I had just begun playing rugby for the school's first fifteen, and had joined the local surf lifesaving club. Now I was reduced to careful swimming – the only sport I could perform that didn't exacerbate the pain.

It was a frustrating time – and also a bit scary,

as I didn't know how much worse it would get or if it would ever improve. I was seventeen years of age, and it seemed crazy that I should be so physically limited at such a young age.

Failed treatments

My pain was first diagnosed as a kneecap mistracking, and I had a considerable amount of physiotherapy to deal with it. However, the problem didn't improve, and eventually I was referred to an orthopedic specialist. The diagnosis was confirmed and he suggested the need to have a look inside with a very small camera (arthroscopy) and release a ligament that was possibly affecting the positioning of the kneecap. Well, that made sense to me and after all he was the expert, so I went ahead with the minor surgery.

Unfortunately there was no improvement postoperatively. At my follow-up, the surgeon had only advice to give but no solutions. The cartilage lining the kneecap had been significantly worn away – an initial sign of arthritis. He advised me to increase my exercise and get into triathlons etc. When I quizzed him on what else could be done, he said the kneecap could be removed!

I left his office feeling quite dejected. I was by then eighteen years of age: I was not about to consider having body parts removed. However, much as I wanted to take up running and cycling again, it was agonisingly painful. More importantly, I figured that if I had already been damaging my joint and had the beginnings of arthritis, wouldn't running make it worse? As far as I could see, if it was that painful, it could be doing more damage.

By this time I was pretty down about the whole situation. It seemed life as I knew it was over. I could no longer run without damaging my knee, so all the things I had taken for granted with sports (other than swimming) I had to stop – as far as I could tell, probably forever! Even sitting with my knees bent for long periods was painful; and something as simple as going to the movies became unenjoyable because of the level of pain involved. So I just had to accept what was happening and do the best I could.

I was in my final year at high school and was deciding what to do when I left. After many sessions at a physiotherapy clinic over the previous year or so, I realised that I had a real interest in how the human body worked. Studying physiotherapy seemed like a logical choice because of this interest, combined with my desire to help others. I worked as hard as I could to get the grades necessary for entry into physiotherapy school.

I ended up on the waiting list, on the chance that someone else decided to pull out. I was obviously being looked after, as a place opened up for me just a few weeks before the physiotherapy school year began.

I had hoped that I might gain more insight to my problem and find a better solution during the four years of study at physiotherapy school. However all I really gained was resignation to the fact that I was 'stuck' with what I had. My long-term prognosis didn't look promising at all.

For my first year out of physiotherapy school I worked at Middlemore Hospital, which was a brilliant teaching hospital, especially for orthopedics. But helping people rehabilitate from knee replacements only really fuelled my lack of hope for my own knees: at this stage, knee replacement was the eventual outcome I would be faced with. This prognosis was depressing – and certainly not the way I wanted things to eventuate!

I refer to 'knees' as plural because by this stage both my knees had become painful. So after six years of this problem I was resigned to a slow deterioration of my knee joints, at best. I was adapting as well as I could: the pain was just bearable when I was cycling, but running was still really painful most of the time.

Finally some hope . . .

To supplement my meagre hospital income I began a job at a private practice down the road from Middlemore. This turned out to be perhaps the best decision I ever made with respect to my knee problem. My boss at the time, Simon Louden, had some new reference books from a course he had just completed, and I began consulting these books when I was a bit 'stuck' on a certain case. Those great reference books were Travell and Simons' *Myofascial Pain and Dysfunction: The Trigger*

Point Manual (Lippincott Williams & Wilkins, 2 vols, 2nd edn, 1998).

One day while I was reading for a particular case I came upon a sentence that strongly resonated with me because of its direct relevance to the pain in my knee. After seven years of getting nowhere, here was a description of a problem that was very similar to mine. The advice the book gave was just to stretch the muscle that was supposedly linked to the aching pain I was getting.

Now this was a little hard to comprehend. Surely the solution couldn't be that simple? After years of physiotherapy, doctors, specialists and surgery with no real benefit, how was I to believe that a simple stretch would help? Not to mention that the joint surfaces were considerably damaged; arthritic changes had begun.

But really, what did I have to lose? At worst, if the stretching made it worse then I would stop.

So I got to stretching. Strangely enough, there was an immediate improvement. The pain level eased slightly, and I could bend my knees a little easier. A small improvement maybe – but this was the first time I had experienced any tangible improvement directly related to treatment! Finally I had a glimpse of hope.

I was now motivated to stretch, which I did relatively regularly over the next few months. Amazingly my knees kept improving. The pain subsided, and I found I could use my knees more and more. Eventually I had no pain to speak of, unless I did a huge amount of exercise and didn't stretch accordingly. What was most incredible, though, was that not only did the aching pain disappear but the sharp pain (like broken glass rubbing under the knee cap) also disappeared! This sharp pain was related to the damage that had been done under the kneecap.

Freedom from pain and stiffness

At this stage I could do anything I wanted physically, without restrictions and certainly with no pain. In fact I was doing things that the specialist had said I would not be able to do and shouldn't do, as it would be too damaging for my knee joint. He was specifically referring to full squats, which put such a huge stress on the joint. However I was able to do these without any pain at all. Even when I added 60 kg onto my shoulders, squatting was still pain-free, and I could squat to the ground and back up again with no problems at all. There was no more of the 'broken-glass' pain under my kneecap. This was incredible, considering that for years prior to this it had been too painful for me to perform a single squat.

Experiencing these changes certainly helped my attitude and outlook on life. However I wasn't entirely convinced that the problems were over: after all, there had been significant damage done to the joint. Time was perhaps the best reassurance; and indeed, my knees have never been bad since. Occasionally I may experience very minor discomfort, but only because I have not been looking after myself – and the discomfort is a great motivator to get back on track.

Putting it to the test

In 2001 I decided to really test how good my knees were. My best mate had encouraged me to team up with him to complete the Speight's Coast to Coast endurance race: my part would be the running and the last cycle leg. I began a year of off-road running and plenty of cycling to prepare the way.

I completed the 33-kilometre run up the Alps, which is mostly rock-hopping up a riverbed. The next day I finished the 70-kilometre cycle to Sumner Beach in Christchurch. By the end of it my knees were still in great shape; the only thing that suffered was my stomach at the thought of having to drink a can of Speight's at the finish line.

My knees felt as good as they had ever felt. I suffered no significant pain, and they were capable of doing everything that they had been able to do before this whole problem started. As far as I was concerned they were as good as ever.

A new perspective in my practice

This whole experience of the last ten years was unfolding as an absolute blessing in my life – not just because the pain and restriction were over, but because it changed my perspective on human anatomy and function. It helped me to reconsider what is happening in all sorts of different muscle and joint pathologies. This in turn has taught me that a lot of what is currently thought to be the cause of certain physical ailments is not necessarily so. More importantly, it has taught me to think and to question what is assumed by most people to be the full answer.

Subsequently I have been able to help people with conditions that may otherwise have been diagnosed as needing either heavy doses of pain relief medication, surgical repair – or were conditions that were just irresolvable.

As a physiotherapist, the blessing has also been how I have been able to relate to people who are experiencing pain and frustration, and how I can help them understand what is going on with their body. Most importantly, I have been able to offer solutions where people had thought there were no answers. I have had the privilege of applying and refining what I have learnt personally into a system that I can apply professionally to many types of physical problems.

Sharing the knowledge

The whole purpose of this book is to share my knowledge with others who can benefit from my experiences and from what I have learned over time. With privilege, I believe, comes responsibility: I have a great desire to share this knowledge to help as many people as possible to enjoy their full physical potential.

I want to be clear that I am not writing this book with the intent of putting down or gainsaying any other health or medical professions or individual practitioners. All areas in healthcare and medicine have plenty of fantastic applications that benefit people in many ways, and I do not want to discredit these great things. However, like all things in this world much can be improved, and I believe I have some answers in this particular area of health.

What I have learned is in my opinion fundamental, and is based on common sense. A lot of the background of what I have studied and researched comes from well documented medical and scientific literature, and much of it has been tested by practitioners and researchers over the last three decades.

What my experience – both personally and professionally – has allowed me to do is to 'connect the dots' and understand at a deeper level what is going on with certain conditions. In the last few years of clinical practice it has become a huge frustration for me to see clients who have been needlessly suffering for months, years, even decades. Often they are taking massive doses of pain-relief medication and anti-inflammatories (sometimes with little relief) that they just don't need if they have an accurate diagnosis and appropriate care.

There is always something that can be done to help people with the conditions outlined in this book – whether it be a modest improvement or complete recovery. More importantly, there is a lot people can do to help themselves, with the right professional guidance. I believe empowering people to be responsible for their own health is a fundamental aspect of all healthcare. My aspiration is to inspire and educate people to do just this.

2

Barking up the wrong tree

An incomplete diagnosis

In my personal and clinical experience, many complications begin from an incomplete diagnosis. Treatments can be ineffective or harmful and may even cause a decline in the person's condition if we are not treating the whole problem. But the most destructive outcome of this is that it can lead to apathy.

People can become resigned to the fact that their condition cannot improve and there is no hope. They give up seeking help, and might live with their condition for months, years, or even a lifetime. Sadly this is all too common, when people could have full resolution of their dysfunction with the correct care. Incorrect diagnosis may result from a health professional jumping to a conclusion because of *some* of the clinical findings.

As health practitioners we can be too quick to rely solely on X-ray, ultrasound and MRI scans. There can be a tendency to assume that these diagnostic 'aids' are the 'be all and end all', whereas in fact we need to use them in conjunction with other diagnostic tools to have a complete picture of what is going on. We can forget to apply common sense with a thorough physical 'hands on' examination. Worse, we sometimes don't use our best diagnostic tool – our ears: listening to clients can give us our best clues. Most problems have *many* contributing factors, but it is too easy to blame the first pathology that we see on X-rays, ultrasound or MRI and ignore what else may be going on.

An example of an incomplete diagnosis

The following case, although it is not osteoarthritis, is a useful example of an incomplete diagnosis.

Jane, a woman in her early fifties, came to see me after suffering for five months with severe lower back pain. She was sleeping only a few hours at a time and was being woken by the pain. She was on high doses of medication but with little relief.

She had been examined by a specialist who had diagnosed her with a disc prolapse, which was detected on MRI. He had given her steroid injections into her back, which gave no relief.

Her prognosis in his opinion was poor and if she didn't improve in the course of the following year he would recommend surgery. He advised that no other treatment would be useful at all.

When I examined her I found severe muscle spasms of her deep lumbar muscles and buttock muscles. After two weeks of treatment her pain was reduced by 50 percent overall. Each time we released some muscle tension she had immediate reduction of pain. Treatment involved massaging her deep spinal muscles and hip muscles with a home stretching regime.

Within a few weeks she was off all painkillers and after about six months she was considerably better. Because she had previously gone for five months with no correct treatment, this case took longer than usual.

I am not denying that prolapse occurred in this case. But it is clear that the disc prolapse was *not the only cause* of pain here. Sometimes what we see on X-ray and scans may have *nothing whatsoever* to do with the client's presenting problem.

3

Why is this not common knowledge?

Misunderstood muscles

I have seen many cases where there has been severe disc prolapse, arthritis, tears and so on, but these have had very little to do with the presenting problem or pain. I am not denying that there are other pathologies present but they may become a 'scapegoat' for the pain when in fact they may not even be causing the actual pain. Sometimes these pathologies have been present for years before the current problem existed.

Why does this happen? In this age of scientific and technological advances how can we get it so wrong?

I believe the primary problem is that there is a major misunderstanding of how the muscular system impacts on our nerves, bones, joints and blood vessels.

The pain that muscles can cause is very misunderstood. Our joints are phenomenal pieces of engineering, but they are governed by the intricate relationship of muscles working together in balance and harmony. If one muscle is not functioning correctly it can completely compromise the whole joint function. This can lead to excruciating pain and, I believe, can possibly even cause severe damage to the joint, much like arthritis.

The effect that muscles have on our bodies is phenomenally underrated, and the far-reaching implications and ramifications they cause often go unnoticed by health practitioners, unless they have specialised experience in this field.

Muscle problems in the neck, for instance, can cause headaches, facial pain, nausea, vomiting, dizziness, and changes in vision. This is well documented. However, almost daily I see people in my clinic who have suffered these problems for months, even years. They have had all sorts of treatments but have often been incorrectly diagnosed and are therefore still stuck with the same problem.

A 'simple' muscle-based problem can result in the most severe pain.

It has been said that muscle-based pain can be as severe as the pain of broken bones.

However, this simple truth of how muscles can affect the body still seems to be largely unaccepted in the wider medical world.

Changes ahead . . .

There is a change towards increasing education in this area: I have seen this over the last 10 years at the School of Physiotherapy at Auckland University of Technology. However, it can take time for mindsets and beliefs to change, and even longer for the follow-on of awareness of this information to filter through to the world at large.

This is my challenge and frustration – and the reason for writing this book. I want to do what I can to help people understand these concepts, and to bring relief to as many people as possible.

My advice to people is to never give up: there is always something that can be done to help. More importantly, find a practitioner who can assess your problem thoroughly and accurately. To do this, the practitioner will need a thorough understanding of how the muscular system can influence nerves, joints and tendons, with specific knowledge of pain referral from muscles.

Here is an example of a person who had suffered from headaches and neck pain for a few years, and who had lost hope and stopped seeking help.

Peter had an X-ray that showed he had severe degeneration to the bones and joints of his neck. Because of this he was advised to stop his work as a farmer and find a new job.

He was frustrated; he was moving less, and putting on weight as a result. Anti-inflammatories were not helping him. He was quite dejected and thought there were no other solutions. He had given up – until he heard about what I was doing with people who had osteoarthritis.

It took one treatment for him to experience relief of his head and neck pain. All I did in this first treatment was to massage the neck muscles, which were extremely tight and tender to touch, until they were a lot freer and less painful. He was astonished to see immediate results.

4

Overlooked causes of pain and stiffness

As I have touched on previously, more often than not the muscular system can be underlying ongoing body pain and other symptoms. Until this is addressed correctly, the problem can continue and may even deteriorate.

Muscle dysfunction can affect the body in many different ways.

Muscles causing pain

Muscles can cause **localised pain** (i.e. pain in the same location as the actual muscle) from muscle spasms or contractions.

Muscles can also cause **referred pain**. This can occur when a muscle spasm or contraction affects nerves that go to other areas of the body. For example, spasms in the trapezius muscle (located in the neck and shoulders) can cause pain into the temple area of the head. This referred pain is the most common cause of misdiagnosis in cases that I see.

The practitioner needs to be aware of *which muscles can refer pain* and *where this pain is referred to*. Otherwise a wrong diagnosis may be made. (As stated previously, Travell and Simons' work on myofascial pain and dysfunction describes this in great detail and is the most comprehensive resource in this area.)

Joint compression

When muscles that cross over a joint are in spasm

or are contracted, they can compress (squash) the joint. The compressive forces produced by muscles in spasm and contraction can be phenomenal.

It is well known that compressive forces can be responsible for wear and tear of joints and possibly for some of the very common degenerative changes associated with osteoarthritis.

As Vic Barker says in *Posture Perfect Doctor*, 'Osteoarthritis is the result of imbalance of muscle tone, and not an inherent disease of the joint.'

These compressive forces can also contribute to other problems, such as disc prolapse. The constant force applied to areas of the spine where there are muscles (in a severely shortened state) attached to it will have an effect on the shape and integrity of the spinal discs.

Those compressive forces will generally irritate the areas that they compress, and this can result in localised inflammation and pain.

Tendon damage and pain

The effects of muscle spasm on tendons can be very severe. This can be seen, for example, in cases of rotator cuff tears.

Ultrasound is the most common way that a tendon tear is diagnosed. Often when a tear is seen there is an immediate conclusion drawn that the tear is what is causing all the pain: case closed.

However, there can be muscle spasm referring pain; and this pain may be referred to exactly the same place where the tendon damage is. This referred pain can be worse than the pain from the actual tendon damage.

Sometimes all the pain is coming from the tight muscle. In these cases, when the muscle spasm is removed the pain can completely disappear (even though the tendon may still be torn!). This further explains why some people have no pain, even though they have damaged or torn tendons. This is a common scenario that I have seen clinically. Furthermore, if the muscle that attaches to a torn tendon is in spasm or is contracted, then it will be adding extra stress and tension to the torn tendon; and in some cases it could be contributing to further tendon damage.

The critical role of muscles in pain and dysfunction

There are several ways we can know that muscles play a critical role in pain and dysfunction. These are explained here.

1. Scientific research and literature

Although in general healthcare and medicine there seems to be little practical understanding of the role of the muscle in pathology, there is a lot of literature and research to validate it. The leading authors in this subject, Drs Travell and Simons, have documented it thoroughly since the 1980s (and Janet Travell had been writing medical papers about the effects of muscle on the body since 1942!). In the first chapter of *Myofascial Pain and Dysfunction* alone there are 300 references to medical papers and texts.

Although there is a need for further scientific study, it is clear that plenty already exists. This existing information first needs to be implemented into mainstream medicine and healthcare.

2. My personal experience

As I said earlier, after suffering from the beginnings of arthritis and finding no answers for seven years, I was able to turn it around in months, just by stretching. This proved to me the value of caring for the muscles – especially when it was evident that there was *already significant damage to the joint*.

3. My clinical experience

In more than fifteen years of applying what I have learned to clients, I have seen countless examples to reinforce the huge part that muscles play in how our body functions. In fact I have seen very few cases where muscles were *not* involved. Sometimes the muscles may contribute only a small amount to the pain, but frequently they are the major contributors.

4. Common sense

I am a practical, down-to-earth person. I believe in common sense and logic. The principles involved with the muscular system as outlined in this book follow logic. For example, if a muscle is in a strong enough spasm it can have an effect on nerves, which can refer pain to another location. When we understand the anatomy of muscles and nerves, this is quite logical.

5. Reproducibility

These areas of pain referral are very similar in nearly all cases. Of course there are a few exceptions, because we are all different in our physical makeup. The case of Mr Scott is a typical example of pain referral.

> Mr Scott thought his hip joint had worn out with OA (osteoarthritis). He had pain deep in the outside aspect of where his hip joint is (i.e. a few inches below the beltline, on the outside of the leg). On examination he had no hip joint problems: his pain was from a deep spinal muscle that can refer pain to this area. When we treated this with pressure release techniques applied to the muscle his pain disappeared.

Here is another good example.

> Mrs Phillips had experienced ongoing pain and problems around her hip joint for more than nine years. Again the deep spinal muscles were the cause, and the problem was resolved after six sessions of pressure point release to the deep spinal muscles.

6. Results

One of the most convincing arguments for the effect of the muscles on the body is the results we get from treatment. It is hard to argue with these, when the original pain and symptoms go away after treatment. It's only logical!

Obviously it is the results that clients want when they come for treatment. When diagnosed accurately and treated correctly and appropriately, then the outcome will be good. That is the reason I found value in this concept initially. It helped me – and it has helped hundreds of people since.

Although the client in the following case study also had a history of rheumatoid arthritis, it is a good example of overlooked causes in the treatment of osteoarthritis.

> Margaret came to see me after suffering with knee pain for over a year. The pain and restriction were getting worse by this stage: she could no longer do her gym workouts and had to stop most of her exercise programmes. When I was assessing Margaret, it was apparent that she didn't really understand what was causing her pain: she seemed unclear and confused. She had been advised that her pain was likely to be

from a previous history of rheumatoid arthritis, and that there wasn't much that could be done to help her.

However, when we rebalanced all her leg muscles with a programme of stretching and massage, she no longer suffered pain and could return to all her previous physical activities. The rebalancing of the muscles allowed the knee joint to function normally again, without the pain and restriction.

5

Inflammation

The Collins English Dictionary defines arthritis as 'inflammation of a joint or joints characterized by pain and stiffness of the affected parts'; and it states that inflammation is characterised by heat, redness, swelling and pain. Herein lies the first problem. The actual definition of OA *implies* inflammation.

If we break the word osteoarthritis down we get the following. Osteo = bone, arthro = joint, and itis = inflammation. This implies also that the bone part of the joint is inflamed.

The misunderstanding created by the literal meaning of the name of osteoarthritis is that inflammation is the primary problem for most cases of OA. This is not always the case and in some cases there will be little or no inflammation. Even in severe cases the inflammation will not always be the primary problem.

Too quickly blamed

As I've said before, the first critical factor in treating joints where there is pain and restriction is a complete and accurate diagnosis. One hurdle in the way of an accurate diagnosis can be the assumption that inflammation is the source of most or all of the pain.

I want to be clear here: I am not claiming that inflammation doesn't cause pain, or that inflammation isn't present in OA. But what I have seen in clinical practice is that inflammation can be blamed as the *main* or *only* cause; other potential causes are not examined or even considered.

I have seen countless examples where clients were using anti-inflammatory medication that would not be helping the pain. When the client stopped taking the medication, their pain was no worse. When such a case improves rapidly without the use of anti-inflammatories, then we have to question how much the inflammation was the cause of the pain in that particular case.

Even when inflammation is present, in some conditions, it may be causing only a very small amount of the pain. Our concern is to accurately find the source or sources of pain, so that we can best deal with the problem.

More possible misunderstandings

While inflammation can be a major factor in OA there are other factors that are also very important. Sometimes the inflammation will be bad; sometimes it will be mild; and sometimes it may even be nonexistent (especially in the less severe cases). However the pain experienced will not necessarily follow the same pattern as the level of inflammation displays. People suffering with OA may have little or no inflammation but still have severe pain.

The other reasons for pain can be joint damage, and muscle problems around the joint.

When we look specifically at OA in this light, some interesting observations can be made with respect to inflammation, muscles and osteoarthritis. This is a major consideration when treating joints with OA. It may sound complicated, but as it unfolds it will become clearer.

A paradox of pain

Here is an example of the apparent paradox frequently observed in OA sufferers. People suffering from osteoarthritis commonly remark that they feel less pain, more comfortable and find it easier to move after having a hot shower or bath. They may also notice that in the cold of winter they are stiffer, and in more pain and discomfort. This is a very common scenario for OA sufferers. This is the crux of the matter.

Remember, with inflammation, 'heat, redness, swelling and pain' are the key factors involved. So to treat inflammation we would use cold to soothe the inflammation: heat would only irritate it. But the opposite occurs a lot of the time. What on earth is going on?

This is where we need to understand the huge effect muscles can have on the joint. Tight, shortened muscles (which are nearly always present in OA) around the affected joint will cause some or all of the pain and stiffness. The hot water will soften and help lengthen these muscles. As the muscle tension eases, the result will be less pain and easier movement.

The opposite usually holds true, too: cold weather or cold applications to the surrounding muscles will result in further contraction or tension in the muscles and can make the pain worse – or at least will not alleviate it.

The exception to this is if the joint involved is inflamed enough for the inflammation to be causing a lot of pain. Then a cold application to the joint will help ease some of the inflammation and thus reduce the pain. In this instance, heat will usually irritate the inflammation and make the pain worse.

Although this is not a conclusive method of testing and diagnosis it does give us some very valuable insight into what is going on. Ideally, when both inflammation and muscles are causing pain, it will help if both hot and cold applications are used appropriately – i.e., cold to the inflamed joint and heat to the tight muscles.

Good news

In my experience I have observed the following:

The more the relief that heating the muscle provides, the more the muscles are contributing to the problem.

This usually means that more can be done to help the problem, using the methods in this book.

'Heating the muscle' means using a moist application of heat (hot-pools, bath, shower, or hot packs soaked in hot water). It does not mean dry heating (using a heat lamp or a wheat bag). Dry heat is better than nothing, but it doesn't get the results that moist heat does.

This is a key factor in understanding the whole problem of OA, and the better you understand it the more you will get out of this system.

> Neil was a thirty-year-old bricklayer. His back had suffered a lot of heavy physical use with his work. He was told that the osteoarthritic changes that had occurred would not respond well to treatment. He reported that he got beneficial effects from a hot spa: his back always felt better after the spa, even after the heaviest days at work. This was a big clue to me that the muscles were involved in his problem.

> Sure enough, when we freed up the lower back muscles with some deep-tissue massage to his deep spinal and hip muscles, the benefits he got were huge and his improvement was dramatic: he stated that he had never had such an improvement with any other treatment. It was interesting that he also reported that with all previous treatment, no one had looked at the muscles we worked on.

I am highlighting this particular point not to discredit other practitioners he had seen, but to illustrate the importance of dealing with the exact muscles that are the issue. If the problem muscles are not dealt with, the result can be no improvement with the pain and stiffness.

6

Bad behaviour

It's not always simple

Muscles are commonly disregarded or overlooked as a major source of pain because their behaviour can be so erratic – and misunderstood. Pain as a result of muscle imbalance confuses people and it can be difficult to see the relationship between the muscle and the pain if some of these principles are not understood.

It is relatively easy to understand how one muscle on its own can cause a problem. When it is treated correctly the problem goes away. However, when the problems are longstanding and there are multiple muscles involved, there are many complications that can arise. This is very off-putting for those who don't understand what is really going on (this is described in detail in the next chapter and the following two chapters, 'Returning pain' and 'Muscle relationships').

Muscle problems are seldom straightforward and simple; in fact, some can be extremely complex. Muscles can have strange and seemingly inexplicable behaviours, which can have odd effects on pain. This is what I call 'bad behaviour'.

Muscles can be in a state of tension and not cause any problems. However, once a certain 'threshold' of tension occurs, the muscle can then cause major pain and suffering. This also applies in reverse: pain can 'disappear' when the muscle tension eases below the threshold.

To confuse matters further, most cases will fluctuate between the states of no pain through moderate pain to severe pain. These extreme changes may occur within a 24-hour period.

This is why sufferers of this type of pain can feel good one day and bad the next, for what seems like no real reason.

This can cause confusion to a practitioner or to a patient who doesn't understand this. The danger is that the real problem will be overlooked.

For a successful outcome the practitioner needs to understand these principles, and also to be able to accurately establish exactly which muscles are involved.

So many variables

There are many factors that will have an impact on the state of tension that the muscle is in. These include:

- **Temperature**: moist heat usually helps, and cold can aggravate the problem. Keeping the muscles protected from cold is essential.

- **Activity and movement/exercise**: some activity or exercise is good, but too much can be detrimental.
- **Repetitive actions**, such as a builder hammering nails all day, or spending hours drilling, can overstress certain muscles.
- **Incorrect posture**: overstressing muscles through bad posture is a particular problem for some people.
- **Prolonged time in any one position**: failing to move around and take the load off certain muscles can lead to overloading of those muscles.
- **Stress**, unconsciously holding tension in one area of the body, or breathing by overusing the accessory neck muscles – as is commonly done when people are stressed – can lead to increased muscle tension.
- **Foods that disagree with your body** (especially for people with allergies), and some foods with chemical additives can have a bad effect on muscle tension.
- **Nutritional status**: a deficiency or lack of certain minerals and vitamins can have a detrimental effect on the state of the muscle.
- **Other pathology/diseases**: some diseases (such as diabetes, thyroid imbalances and

adrenal fatigue) can irritate muscles.

- **Medications**: cholesterol-lowering drugs, for example, are known to have some side effects on muscles.

Not all of these factors may be relevant in all cases, but they need to be considered, especially if things do not improve as they should.

If any of these factors are present and are not addressed then the success of the treatment can be limited.

Temperature

Moist warmth eases muscle tension, so I advise keeping the muscles warm with appropriate warm clothing. Soaking in hot water, e.g. hot-pools, bath or shower, is the best method to ease muscle tension. Mud packs are also very good. Dry heat such as wheat bags, hot-water bottles etc are useful but tend to be not as effective as hot-water applications.

Conversely, cold applications will normally cause muscle tension to increase. This is why we advise caution with ice – and limit it to only inflamed areas.

The effect of heat and cold on the muscle is why we have the paradox that I described earlier with reference to inflammation.

Exercise and movement

Exercise that involves blood pumping through the muscles will result in 'heating' of the muscles (Michael J Alter, *Sport Stretch*, 2nd edition, 1998). If the OA isn't too severe, people may feel their joints are freer and less painful once they have warmed up with exercise, especially if it is not heavy, jarring exercise. However, repetitive movements of problem areas can irritate and overload some muscles and make the problem worse. The ideal is to find the balance so that people keep moving without overdoing it physically and overworking their problem muscles. This is described in more detail in the next chapter.

Posture

Poor posture that puts excess stress on particular muscles will often result in an increase in muscle tension in certain areas – as will repetitive activities, especially if they are performed with poor posture. A typical example is someone with neck pain who has poor head and neck posture. For many people, poor posture involves the person's head jutting forward relative to their neck, instead of keeping it in line with the shoulders and the chin tucked. This 'chin jut' posture puts stress on the muscles at the back of the neck.

Poor posture can also be seen in poor walking patterns due to incorrect movement in the back and hip, or foot and ankle. Poor footwear can cause this. One very common problem with footwear is raised heels. Contrary to common belief, even a very low heel can be detrimental to the posture and hence the state of the muscles. In his book *Posture Makes Perfect*, Dr Vic Barker explains that heels change the position of the spine, hip, knee and ankle joints; this in turn alters the normal function of all the associated muscles.

Stress

Emotional stress can add to muscle tension. This can be alleviated by relaxation exercises, and by learning and practising correct breathing habits (Bradley et al.).

Poor breathing can have a direct effect on the neck muscles. Ways to improve this may be found in the DVD on treating the neck. This DVD is in my complete system of treatment. There is also a CD with a guided relaxation exercise in the system to help people deal with stress. If you don't have the system, you can find out more at www.freedomfromarthritis.com.

Nutritional status

The impact of nutrition on muscle function is a large topic in its own right and is beyond the scope of this book. However, it is worth noting the following here.

Calcium, magnesium, iron and potassium are minerals that can affect muscles. Vitamins C, B1, B6 and B12 can also affect muscles. There are many books that explain such things. For more detail on this, see Travell and Simons' *Myofascial Pain and Dysfunction*; and see the 'Further reading' section at the end of this book.

If the muscles are not responding to normal treatment, it may be worth investigating a person's nutritional status. Eating foods rich in these nutrients or taking supplements can be useful but there may be other factors affecting the absorption of these, including other pre-existing health issues.

Some food and drink – such as coffee, alcohol and chocolate – can require extra vitamins and minerals for them to be processed in the body. So in some cases eating and drinking these foods can deplete the body of the vitamins and minerals that it needs to maintain muscle health.

Many so-called 'foods', such as junk food, can have a harmful effect on the state of tension of the muscular system too. Monosodium glutamate (MSG) has been linked to neck pain and headaches

(see Bill Statham, *The Chemical Maze*).

Other pathologies

There may also be other pathologies affecting the body that we can't ignore. All health factors must be considered, especially if there are other health problems that can affect the joints and pain. Thyroid problems and adrenal fatigue have been shown to contribute to problems of the muscles (see Dr James Wilson, *Adrenal Fatigue*) Hypoglycaemia (low blood sugars) and diabetes can also have an effect on the state of the muscles (Travell and Simons).

Medications

Certain medications may also have side effects that can affect the muscles; these should be discussed with your doctor. Cholesterol-lowering medications are known for their effect on muscles. Beatrice Golomb MD, PhD, Associate Professor of Medicine at the University of California, San Diego School of Medicine has co-authored a paper on the adverse effects of statins, published in the online edition of *American Journal of Cardiovascular Drugs*. She states, 'Muscle problems are the best known of "statin drugs"' adverse side effects'.

All of the above factors must be addressed when dealing with muscles, especially when putting all the information together in a case; then we can accurately draw conclusions as to what is going on.

Until the muscles return to normal they will be

prone to these fluctuations in pain. It can take months to achieve a balanced state.

When the muscles are behaving

The key message to take out of this is the importance of maintaining the muscles around an affected joint in an optimal length, with little or no muscle tension. When this state is maintained and achieved the best outcome can be realised. The following case illustrates how returning the muscles to normal even when OA is present can result in pain elimination.

> Mrs Townsend (75) came to see me after being involved in a motor vehicle accident about six weeks earlier. As it turned out she had OA in her thumbs but had had no problems with this prior to the accident; in fact she didn't even know she had OA.
>
> I had sent her for an X-ray to check she didn't have any broken hand or wrist bones. The X-ray showed some longstanding OA (but thankfully no breaks).

Some health professionals might assume that the OA was irritated by the accident and that there would be little that could be done to help. However, I assessed her hands, wrists and forearms and found some interesting results: her thumb muscles were in terrible spasm.

When her muscle tension was resolved her pain was no longer an issue. Furthermore her problem was resolved with minimal treatment from me (three sessions of pressure point release) and her own home stretching programme.

The best part was that as we returned the problematic muscles back to normal her pain disappeared.

This is such a good example as it shows how huge a factor the muscles play, even in a case where OA is present.

7

Returning pain

Failure and frustration

One of the frustrating aspects of pain caused by muscles is how it can disappear and then return again. This can be devastating for the sufferer.

In the majority of straightforward cases this 'returning pain' should cease once the case is dealt with completely. However, if the 'returning pain' is not addressed then there is a real danger of failure. The reason for this is twofold.

The sufferer may not at first recognise the benefits of the immediate treatment. With time, explanation and reassurance this can be addressed so that they begin to understand and accept the process.

However, if the sufferer doesn't understand the process, they may become dejected and stop the course of treatment. I have seen many cases (especially in my early years of practice) where this has occurred. Unfortunately it can mean the end of what might otherwise have been a very successful outcome.

I believe this is so critical that I have spent a lot of time in this area, in clinical practice, to prevent it happening wherever possible. This is also why I have dedicated a whole chapter to the subject.

Many patients, after the first or second treatment, have said to me, 'The treatment is not working; I am no better now than I was when I first came to see you.' But while they may not be any better (or only slightly better) at that moment in time, most of the time they would have experienced massive improvements immediately after the treatment. These improvements may have only been temporary but they may well have been an indicator that there is a huge potential for resolution of their problem.

Here is a good example of this situation.

> Mrs Gregory (87) came to see me with moderate osteoarthritis in her knees. She was in a reasonable amount of pain,

especially walking up and down stairs. She was having trouble with her balance and was feeling that her legs were weak and unstable. Her knee muscles were in a terrible state of imbalance and would benefit from some treatment.

After her second treatment she left the clinic and could walk up and down the stairs with none of the knee pain that she had experienced. This improvement lasted for the next few days, and even her son commented that she was walking better and didn't need her walking stick. However the pain returned after about a week (just prior to her next appointment). Because the pain had returned, she thought the treatment had failed.

On examination, the muscles that we had previously released had tightened up again. We released the muscles and explained this process of the muscles tightening up again. She left and walked down the stairs again without pain.

She was quite discouraged as the pain kept 'returning', and she needed lots of reassurance and encouragement to keep her on track with treatment. After all, she had been suffering with the problem for over ten years and it was going to take time to get the best result.

There are two main issues to deal with in respect to returning pain.

1. Muscles that are problematic around a joint need to be fully released to return to a normal state.

2. Other contributing factors need to be identified and addressed (and removed where possible).

Releasing the muscle

Fully restoring the muscles to their normal state can take a considerable amount of time, especially in cases where the muscles have been out of balance for many years. If the muscles are not fully restored to their normal state, this can result in the pain returning over and over again.

The treatment should continue until the pain and problems are resolved. However, in some severe cases of OA where there is severe degeneration of the joint, the problem may improve but never fully be resolved. In these cases ongoing treatment will probably be necessary to maintain the best level of success. This is where using a home-based self-treatment programme can be of huge benefit.

Other contributing factors

The most common factors that need to be addressed with regard to returning pain are posture and activity.

There are many misconceptions around muscle use and abuse. Balance is critical with respect to health, and with reference to muscle activity the concept of balance is paramount. Too little movement will result in seizing up and weakness of muscles. On the other hand, too much activity and overloading the muscles, combined with insufficient self-care (i.e. stretching, massage, heat and gentle movement), can be equally detrimental – and is much more common.

I often hear patients say, 'I haven't been doing

much exercise lately so that is why my muscles are so tight.' However, the muscle tension they are experiencing is more likely due to the fact that they have overloaded the area and haven't stretched enough to counteract the use the muscles have had.

Exercise and activity

What constitutes too much exercise or activity is specific to each individual case. Common sense needs to be applied, taking into account the severity of each case. If there are doubts then professional advice should be sought in this area.

Generally speaking movements and activity should be gentle, deliberate and made cautiously. Any activities requiring heavy lifting, sustained lifting, sustained positions or repetitive activities should be avoided where possible during the treatment. This is especially important at the beginning of the treatment, when the effects of the treatment are being assessed.

When the muscle has returned to its normal state, or has made significant improvement, then gradual and careful activities can be reintroduced over a period of time. If there is any deterioration when the activities are reintroduced, they will need to be stopped and reintroduced more slowly once things have settled down again.

The golden rule is not to exercise to the point where muscles are becoming fatigued.

The same principles apply to what might be considered 'easy' activities, such as driving a vehicle for more than 20 minutes, walking for more than 15 minutes, standing in one position for over 15 minutes or sitting for over 30 minutes. Although these may seem easy, they may cause muscle fatigue, which can lead to poor posture and overloading of muscles.

The idea is to get you thinking about how you are using your body, and to vary the position you perform activities in – while maintaining good posture and body awareness – to make them as easy as possible.

More on Posture

Poor posture that puts excess stress on particular muscles can result in an increase in muscle tension in certain areas. Likewise, repetitive activities, especially if they are performed with poor posture, can cause muscle stress.

An example of poor posture is when someone stands with their body inclined forward and their head jutting forward of their body. In this position, the muscles at the back of the legs and the muscles of the spine will be working excessively just to keep them upright (Kendall et al, *Muscles: Testing and Function, with Posture and Pain*).

People may not consider sleep an activity, but incorrect body positioning during sleep can put added stress on some muscles which can cause further problems. Correct pillow height and a suitable mattress are critical to a good sleeping posture. (Note that specific individual advice on this is beyond the capacity of this book;

professional help is recommended if this is an issue, e.g. from a physiotherapist, osteopath or occupational therapist.)

Failure to address all the factors of muscle behaviour explained above can lead to complete confusion of what is really responsible for the pain. I have seen cases with some clients who had come to see me after being told that their pain was 'in their head', because the previous practitioner didn't understand, or didn't explain clearly, what was going on. One case was so extreme that the patient was referred to a psychiatrist for his pain – when in fact the pain was from a neck muscle imbalance.

With appropriate treatment, the pain should keep going away after each session. Also, improvement should last longer after each session. This sequence usually means that the outcome and prognosis are positive.

Once the problems of the 'returning pain' are identified and understood, there are specific actions that can be taken to reduce and rectify its occurrence. This is where an appropriate programme is needed, not only to address the immediate muscle tension but also to prevent the muscle from returning to a state of tension again.

Application of heat, stretching and self-massage techniques are all very useful for achieving this. After this, the 'normal' state of the muscle can be resumed so that the problem won't continue. These are discussed in specific detail in chapter 11 'Restore'.

8

Muscle relationships – the curve ball

Just when you think you are getting to grips with all the ways muscles can cause pain, you get thrown a curve ball: the pain moves.

The relationships between various muscles are a big factor to consider when dealing with OA. Misunderstanding these relationships can result in confusion and an unsatisfactory outcome. Treating OA (especially if it has been present for some time) can be similar to peeling an onion: as we remove one muscle issue there can be other muscle problems underneath.

There are two things to be aware of with respect to muscle relationships.

1. The pain may move around from place to place (especially after a particular muscle or muscle group has been released).

2. Each muscle or group of muscles around a joint can affect the other muscles of that joint.

Changing pain locations

With osteoarthritis there can be several muscles under tension at one time. However, when we examine someone with pain there may be one particular muscle that is causing most of the pain. When this particular muscle has been released it should no longer cause the pain it had been causing. However, it is possible that one of the other muscles that was previously under tension now causes pain elsewhere. The exact location of the new pain will be determined by which muscle is under tension.

This is a process of 'rebalancing' the muscles so that they can *all* return to their normal state of functioning. In complex or longstanding cases, many muscles may be involved. For example in lower back pain there can be up to nine different muscles involved.

Sometimes the muscles involved may be right next to each other, so when each muscle is released the pain may shift location by only a few millimetres. Other times the muscles may be opposite each other at a joint: this will usually result in the pain going to the other side of the joint. The following case illustrates how the pain can change location as the different muscles come into play.

Mrs Ascot, aged seventy-six, came to see me with severe OA of her knee. The pain was mostly in the front of her knee. Each time we released the muscles in the front of her knee the pain would leave the front of her knee. Her knee movement would increase immediately – but she would then experience the pain at the back of her knee as we moved the knee further. We would then release the muscles in the back of her knee and, as a result, she would lose the pain at the back of her knee and her movement would increase again. But the pain would return to the front of the knee as we moved the knee further.

The pain kept alternating as we released the muscles of the front and back of the knee, and the knee gained more and more movement.

The point here is that the outcome was good – i.e. we were significantly improving movement in her knee. The changing pain is an indication of what is happening to the muscles, and the effect that the muscles are having on the joint.

However, if the sufferer does not understand this process, then these changes can be misunderstood. The sufferer may think that no good is resulting from the treatment, in spite of the fact that movement is improving right before their eyes. This can be a time when people 'give up', thinking they can't be helped.

I want to highlight this example so people can understand as much as possible about what is happening, so that they do not lose hope when things may overall be actually improving. When the process is understood the appropriate treatment can follow and the best results can be achieved.

Altered muscle function and the joint

Although some muscle imbalances may not cause direct pain, they can be responsible for abnormal movement of a joint. This can result in extra demands and stress on other muscles of that joint. Damage, inflammation and wear and tear around that joint can then follow. The following case is an example of this.

> Ernest (38) had pain up by his elbow, on the outside of his forearm. The pain was coming from his forearm muscles on the same side of his arm. But the muscles on the other side

of his forearm were causing stress on the problem muscles, so these muscles also needed to be released.

The important consideration here is that all the muscles of a joint are balanced so that good quality movement can be achieved, and there is no unnecessary wear and tear to our joints.

9

Review

Three fundamental steps

Over the last fourteen years I have fine-tuned my system of treating osteoarthritis and have simplified it to three fundamental steps:

Review, Record and Restore.

Each step is critical in this order to get the best results possible in the shortest space of time and with the best understanding of the process. The Review step is discussed in detail in this chapter, the Record step is discussed fully in chapter 10, and the Restore step is detailed in chapter 11.

Reviewing all relevant information

The process of reviewing means gathering all the relevant information with respect to your osteoarthritis. This includes the following:

1. Pain pictures
2. Radiological examination, X-ray, ultrasound, MRI, CT scan

Physical Examination
3. General appearance of the joint
4. Joint movement
5. Muscle movement
6. Muscle tension

This is the first step in this method of treatment. Read through this chapter and answer the following questions to complete the review process. As you go it is essential to record your findings: this is described in detail in the next chapter. I suggest reading chapter 10 before completing the questions outlined below.

Creating a pain picture

The first step in the reviewing process is to create a 'pain picture'. This is often the most time-consuming part of the whole assessment process, but it is essential for gathering all relevant information. I use the prompts *what*, *where*, *when*, *why* and *how* as a guide.

How does the pain feel? Is the pain an ache, a sharp pain, burning pain or another type of pain?

How intense is the pain? A useful method for grading this is by using a scale from 0 to 10, where 0 refers to no pain at all and 10 is the worst pain you have ever experienced. As a rough guide, a pain rating of 2–3 is more an annoyance than a real hindrance; 5 is moderate (more than just annoying pain); 7 is quite severe and will be inhibiting some activities such as physical activities and sleep.

If there is more than one type of pain you will need to grade each different pain.

Where exactly is the pain? It is useful to note this

exactly, not just 'my knee hurts' – for example, 'my knee hurts underneath the kneecap' or 'at the back to the left'. Again, if there is more than one pain, pinpoint exactly where each pain is.

This step is very important as the treatment progresses and the pain may move (see chapter 8).

When does it hurt? Often people will say their pain is continuous, but when we look at it closely it isn't (though it may seem like it to them, especially when they have had it for a long time). It is critical to understand when exactly the pain comes and goes, when it eases and when it gets worse. To treat the problem, we also need to know when the pain began; whether there were any relevant injuries, and so on.

If there is more than one type of pain we need to know exactly when each pain occurs.

What makes the pain worse, and what makes it better? Here, think about elements that exacerbate or relieve the pain, such as heat or cold, exercise, rest or sleep.

What can you not do because of the pain?
What activities can you no longer perform because of the pain? Include daily activities around the

house (e.g. hanging out the washing, walking up the stairs, gardening, etc).

What other things can you no longer do due to the pain? (e.g. sports and recreation).

List everything you can think of, as some of these activities may become easier and this will help you identify your progress in time to come.

What drugs do you have to take, how often and when?

I suggest keeping a diary as a record: you can enter details each day to get a good idea of what is going on. It is amazing what patterns show up, and also what connections are made with respect to possible contributing factors and causes of the pain.

Radiological examination

Radiological examination using MRI, X-ray, ultrasound etc can be very useful to determine what we can't see inside the joint. However, on its own with no other considerations, it is only one piece of the puzzle. If you have had X-rays or similar then you should have a report to go with these. This is useful as a summary of what the X-rays show, so that it makes some sense to you.

If there is no summary it would pay to have the X-rays read by someone who is qualified and experienced to do this.

Physical Examination

General Appearance

We gain valuable information when we consider the external appearance of the joint. We are looking especially for signs of inflammation: redness, heat, swelling, shape and alignment of the joint. This is more obvious for some joints such as ankles, elbows or hands; and less obvious for deeper joints such as hips and spine.

Joint movement

Movement of the joint is very important. Here we look at how much movement the joint has compared with what it normally should have; and also how the joint feels with movement. Usually we will measure the problem joint against a normal joint though this is difficult if both joints are affected! For most people, this is a skill you will need more specific help with. It is explained in the instructional DVDs that I have compiled as part of my entire system for self-management of osteoarthritis.

Muscle movement

It is critical to assess and measure the amount of movement of each muscle that affects the joint. This is a skill that you will need more specific help with. It is explained in detail in the instructional DVDs.

Muscle texture

The muscle must be examined physically to look at muscle tension and pressure points. Here we are looking not just at how tight the muscles feel but also where the painful parts of the muscle are and how intense the pain is with pressure on these points. Usually, the more painful these points are and the tighter the muscles are is proportional to the amount of potential for improvement.

Once again, this is a specific skill that you will need help to use. It is further explained in the accompanying instructional DVDs, or visit www.freedomfromarthritis.com to access all the tools to help yourself.

The most common problem I see is that some cases are not fully examined.

Paul was a sixty-year-old man who had been told he had osteoarthritis of his knees and there was nothing that could be done. This diagnosis had been given after only an X-ray and with no thorough physical examination of his joints and muscles.

While we were discussing his problem (creating his pain picture) it became evident to me that he was likely to have some problems with his front hip and knee muscles. Sure enough, when we examined these muscles they were in a dreadfully tight state.

I performed four sessions of massage and stretching these muscles, and he took on a stretching regime to finish the treatment.

He was amazed at the outcome. He could comfortably ride a bike and run without being stopped by pain. He had thought he would never do these activities again as they had been so painful.

After completing the review stage we are formulating a more complete picture of the OA and this helps us to move on to the next step of recording this information.

10

Record

Why record the information?

Recording the information from the review process may seem like a trivial and unimportant step to some people. However I have noticed in many cases that it is paramount to the success of the treatment, and has proven to be one of the most fundamental areas to address.

In my clinical practice I record all clinical details during a patient's initial assessment and with subsequent follow-ups. Of course we keep notes for professional reasons and as a legal requirement, but we also keep notes to achieve the highest possible outcome. The same holds true for this system of treatment at home. This process is creating a comprehensive baseline of where you are at right now, so that you will have a clear idea of your progress as the treatment continues.

As I hope you have gathered, this is not a quick-fix solution to your problem but a comprehensive system that will give you tools to help yourself over a period of time. Sure there are some cases that will improve in a very short space of time, but this is not the expected outcome for everyone. Some OA sufferers may have had problems for years and undoing some of the related issues can take many months.

Being aware of and recording your progress through the treatment will help you to see improvements – even if they are small – which will greatly help you to stay motivated and committed to the treatment that is best suited to your condition. Furthermore this will allow the most accurate feedback on your progress, so that the best course of treatment can be realised.

How to record

It is important to record the information as concisely and clearly as possible so that it is clear and easy to refer to. This is why I have compiled the workbooks that accompany this book and the DVDs on the system. All these resources are available from the website at www.freedomfromarthritis.com, if you don't have copies of all of them.

Workbook #1 is where you can input all your answers that you develop from the review process in chapter 9. Ideally, it would be best to write your answers into the relevant spaces in the workbook at the time that you answer these questions.

As mentioned in the previous chapter, this book does not contain all the information to accurately complete all of the physical examination. Trying to clearly explain how to perform the examination in a book alone would be very difficult. This is why I have compiled the DVDs, as a tool to guide you through the rest of the physical examination in this review phase (as well as the tools for complete treatment techniques) for each joint covered in the system. The idea is that you can then perform the examination yourself at home; or, if you need help from a suitable health practitioner, you will understand more about the process.

Workbook #2 is to keep ongoing records after you begin the treatment. This can then be compared to your baseline records to help measure your progress over time.

The information in the workbooks and on the DVDs is critical for completing the self-treatment programme. If you don't have these, they can be accessed at www.freedomfromarthritis.com.

Other benefits of keeping a record

There are other reasons as to why recording this information is so useful:

- It will help you understand your problem more clearly, and this clarity is highlighted when it is written down on paper, not just 'left in your head'.

- It can be quite a revelation when it is written down, as it can 'sink in' deeper and makes more sense.
- And, of course, if it is written down then it won't be forgotten!

Once you have a complete picture of where your problem is at present, you will be ready to move on to the next phase of the system. This is the restore phase, where the 'treatment' part of the system is explained.

As I mentioned earlier, I always record all details when I see clients in practice as this is critically valuable. The benefits of this can be seen in the following case.

> Mr Lee (62) was suffering from pain on the inner aspect of his knee, and had just had minor surgery with a cartilage (meniscus) repair. His pain was no better post surgery, and he was advised that the only option left was to have a knee replacement.
>
> Examination of his knee showed that he had excellent joint movement, but a problematic muscle that attached to the area of his knee was painful. Over the course of three treatments, things were improving steadily but not quite resolving as expected.
>
> I had kept detailed notes of what was

happening, so I noticed a small anomaly: the pain returned each time after he played a round (18 holes) of golf. This may seem obvious – but he was fine after playing nine holes. The difference was the added walking, which was exacerbating the problem. So to compensate I suggested he increase the stretching before and after the 18-hole games. After two more follow-up consultations he was ok after playing 18 holes, and no longer had any problems.

If I had not kept detailed notes, it could have been easy to miss this critical detail and fail to get a satisfactory result.

11

Restore

What you can do

This is the 'how to' section of the book, where you will get the information to help you to overcome your pain. However, if you've jumped straight to this chapter without reading the previous chapters, then you will have missed some critical parts. Just like baking a cake, if you skip some of the initial steps (like leaving out some ingredients or not mixing it properly) then you will have a pretty sad cake at the end of it. It is important to do this properly if you want to get the best results. So you don't waste your own time: invest the time in yourself and give yourself the best chance of helping yourself. You deserve it.

There are of course other considerations when treating OA – such as dealing with inflammation, poor posture, damage to joints, poor biomechanics. But the key element of this present method is restoring the muscles to as close to normal as possible, and keeping them that way.

Stretching the muscle

There are various methods to help restore the muscles. Essentially, they are all a form of stretching.

Most people think of stretching as putting the body into a particular position to stretch a particular muscle, such as pulling your heel to your buttock to stretch your front thigh muscles. This is of course true, but there are other ways of stretching that are also very effective.

- **Massaging** is one way in which we can stretch a muscle – either by working over the whole muscle or on a particular part of the muscle.
- **Pressure point (trigger point) release** is another way the muscle can be stretched.
- **Heat** applied to the muscle doesn't stretch the muscle as such, but it does help it to relax and stretch more effectively.

Can releasing the muscles around joints with OA actually help in any real significant way? In all the cases I have ever seen, the muscles around the joint with OA were in an altered state of tension. The message is simple.

The worse the state of tension the muscles are in, the greater the potential for improvement.

If there is little damage to the joint, or if the damage doesn't cause any restriction in joint movement, then the potential for improvement is even greater. This assumes, of course, that there are no other pathologies involved.

Nearly all cases improve and some are completely resolved (meaning the person can achieve full movement and use with no pain). If there is a great amount of joint damage and inflammation then the results may not be as good, but even in the worst cases there can be a significant decrease in pain and increase in movement. Of course there are some severe cases that have no improvement at all, but these are very few.

The level of success that can be attained is only fully known after these methods have been applied correctly and consistently over a period of time.

Where to start

Knowing where to begin with the treatment can be difficult, especially if you haven't completed the review and record steps in chapters 9 and 10. As explained previously, Review, Record and Restore need to be done in order, as each step follows the other.

While reviewing the muscle movement and joint

movement (outlined in chapter 9 and detailed in the DVDs and on the website) it is likely that you will have seen some restriction in one or both movements. Basically, if you can put the muscle into a stretched position and not hurt or irritate the joint, then you will probably be able to begin stretching immediately – so long as there is no increase in joint pain.

If it is clear that the stretching is causing an increase in joint pain, then it would be unwise to continue until it is more comfortable to stretch. In some cases there are modifications to the stretch that can reduce or remove the pain. These are described in the DVDs for each joint. However, if the modified stretches are still too painful then stretching should be avoided until there is improvement.

If this is the case there are other techniques that can be useful, such as pressure point release or massage, which shouldn't irritate the joint if performed correctly. These techniques typically produce more immediate improvements than passive stretching does. The improvements from these techniques can also be more obvious and may be seen quite quickly compared with what may be seen with stretching. By all means, if you have the resources, you can begin right away with the massage or pressure point release techniques, as they can speed up recovery time.

Let's get specific about each of these techniques.

Self (passive) stretching

This technique is brilliant, as it can be performed solely by the individual themselves. The downside is that, in some cases, pain and restricted movement will limit its usefulness. Don't despair, though, if you can't stretch the first time you try. With some massage or pressure point releasing, the ability to stretch may improve over time. Try those other techniques for a few weeks first until things improve, then try stretching again.

When I was stretching for my knee problem, I would often have to stop because of knee pain (the 'broken-glass' feeling under my kneecap). But I found that by altering my positioning or waiting for it to settle I could continue at another time.

Having a little bit of discomfort stretching is

usually okay. The rule is, it should feel better (and certainly not more painful) after stretching. If it feels worse afterwards, then stop and try another time. 'Pushing through' pain can be harmful as it can irritate and damage joints. If in doubt seek advice from an appropriate health practitioner.

How to stretch

I have seen many misconceptions around stretching over the last twenty years in the health field. I believe the reason is that there are so many different forms of stretching – from the gentle, passive stretches to the vigorous ballistic stretches, and everything in between. In addition, there are so many factors that affect the state that the muscles are in (see chapter 6 'Bad behaviour').

For the purposes of this book I am specifically referring to **passive stretching** only. Passive stretching is moving the involved limb gently to the end of its movement, until a moderate stretching sensation is felt in the muscle. When the stretch is felt, hold that position for 30 seconds, keeping as still as possible.

This stretch should be performed carefully and smoothly, with no bouncing, jerking or forcing. Pain should be avoided. However, with an effective stretch there will be a sensation of moderate discomfort in the muscle being stretched.

While you hold the position for 30 seconds (assuming pain does not begin during this time), it is helpful to perform relaxed, slow breathing while focusing on relaxing all muscles that are not being used. During the exhalation (breathing out), a good practice is to consciously relax the muscle being stretched as much as possible.

It is a good idea to use a clock or stopwatch to time the 30-second duration: this leaves you free to focus on maintaining the correct stretching technique.

After each stretch, move the joint out of the stretch position and through its full range of movement a few times.

Each muscle should be stretched a minimum of three times at each stretching session (assuming there is no increase in pain). Ideally this regime of three stretches for 30 seconds should be repeated three times over a day – a suggestion is to stretch after waking, during the day and before bed at night. If you are engaged in any physical activity or are in one position for long periods during the day, you may well need to stretch more to alleviate the aggravations these activities can cause.

Stretching is always easier when the muscle is warm; however in most cases it is not necessary to go for a 5-minute jog or to take a hot bath prior to stretching. If the stretching is performed gently, as described above, it should not cause any harm. Pain is always the best guide to avoiding damage. In some cases where stretching under normal conditions would be too painful, soaking in a hot bath or shower may help to make the stretch less painful.

Pain relief medications may mask the normal awareness of pain. For this reason, extra care must be taken so that you do not overdo the stretch. If in doubt, seek appropriate medical advice before stretching.

A good, well performed stretch may be uncomfortable to start with, but by the end of the stretching procedure the discomfort should have eased considerably. If it has not eased then the stretch is either:

- applied too strongly
- performed incorrectly, or
- there may be another problem such as joint damage limiting movement.

Pressure point or trigger point release

Of all the techniques to 'stretch' the muscle this is the safest with respect to not aggravating the joint.

Safety first

There are some specific safety issues when it comes to applying pressure to certain areas of the body, and for your safety these need to be addressed. It is strongly advisable if you need to work over these areas that you get a safety clearance from a medical practitioner so that you can do this safely. The reason for this is that if there are pre-existing blood clots or plaque build-up in these areas, deep pressure/massage could result in moving these clots and causing serious complications, some of which could be fatal.

If you need to be applying pressure or massage to the side of the neck or the groin or the back of the knee or calf muscle, then you should ask a doctor for the okay to do so first.

Finding the trigger points

First, you need to find the trigger points for the muscles surrounding the affected joint. Pressure is then gradually applied onto that point, using a finger or thumb. Other items such as a tennis ball or a jack knobber can be used to apply extra pressure, especially for difficult areas to reach, e.g. buttocks or shoulder-blade muscles.

When pressure is applied in the correct spot it will usually be painful, but this tenderness should reduce to a much lower level after a minute or two. In some cases where the muscle has been very tight for a long period of time, the pain doesn't reduce much initially: a gentler approach may be needed.

If the pain doesn't reduce at all or just gets worse, medical advice should be sought to check there are no other causes of pain.

Some muscles have many of these pressure points, and these should all be worked in the same manner. When the technique is successful, the points will be less tender to touch and the joint should feel easier to move. Pain should also decrease. All muscles around the joint need to be released, especially if the area of pain changes after one muscle group has been released (see chapter 8 on muscle relationships and changing pain locations).

Massage

Massage is another very effective way of reducing muscle tension, but for some areas it is quite difficult to do effectively on yourself. If you have the resources to get a professional massage this can be a good way to help.

Safety

The same specific safety issues apply for massage to certain areas of the body as for pressure point release (see above). For your safety, these need to be addressed. It is strongly advisable if you need to work over these areas that you get a safety clearance from a medical practitioner first. The reason for this is that if there are pre-existing blood clots or plaque build-up in these areas deep pressure/massage could potentially result in moving these clots and causing serious complications, some of which could be fatal.

If you are applying pressure or massage to the side of the neck, the groin, or the back of the knee or calf muscle, you should ask a doctor for the okay to do so first.

The other consideration here is with respect to inflammation of joints. Heavy or deep massage on a joint that is inflamed is not a good idea. It can irritate and increase inflammation. A few very gentle flowing strokes over an inflamed joint may help the inflammation, but keep the deep, heavy strokes to the bulk of the muscle and avoid any heavy pressure on or close to inflamed joints.

Where to apply massage?

Massage will need to be applied over the whole affected muscle, and to all the muscles that surround the joint being treated. With effective massage the muscles will feel less tight/hard to the person massaging, and the result should be easier movement and less pain in the involved joint.

For maximum effectiveness the whole muscle needs to be fully released. In cases that have been present for a long time this may take quite a few sessions of massage to get significant changes.

How often should massage or pressure point release be administered?

How often you should administer massage or pressure point release is determined by two factors.

1. **How much the person can handle.** Some people can handle up to 1 hour of deep pressure tissue treatment every day. Others can tolerate only one short session of light pressure every 3–4 days. If in doubt, the advice is to start gently (not too deep pressure), and leave at least 24 hours in between the massage sessions – assuming it is not too tender to touch after this time.

2. **How much the person needs.** In mild cases, one session a week may be all that is needed. Moderate cases may need a couple of sessions a week, while severe cases may need up to three sessions per week – if the muscles are not too sore from the work done.

The frequency of treatment is gauged by how long the benefit lasts for. Assuming there was a reduction or elimination of pain, it is ideal to repeat the treatment as the pain increases again – but only if the muscles worked on are not too tender. Often a day or two in between treatments is necessary.

When beginning the treatment, more regular sessions are most useful. I would see someone two to three times a week for the first two to three weeks to get the best results, assuming it was effective and there was good progress. Once the improvement lasts longer I increase the time between sessions; this can be anywhere from once a week to once a month.

You need to be mindful of any pain relief or anti-inflammatory medications that you may be using. These may mask the pain that you would normally have, which could result in you pushing your movement to a level that could be damaging but that you don't feel because of the medications.

It is advisable to seek medical help to be safe in this instance.

What to expect

You may remember what my experience was when I began stretching for my knee pain (back in chapter 1): I noticed that my pain reduced slightly after the first set of stretches and my movement was a bit less painful and also freer.

This reaction is pretty typical: it was not a miracle cure, where I could have immediately run up a flight of stairs pain-free; just a noticeable improvement, with pain easing slightly and movement increasing slightly. Sure, in some cases the result is immediate and full, but this does not happen for everyone. Usually, the milder the degree of OA the quicker and better the immediate change; and conversely, the more severe the OA the slower and less obvious the change. But if I hadn't persevered for a few months I wouldn't have got the great results I did.

As long as this method of treatment gives you some relief (and doesn't increase pain) the absolute key is committing to following the instructions as closely as possible for as long as it takes to achieve the best outcome. As in my case it could take many months to do this.

In the more severe cases people may not be able to stretch without irritating the joints. Where this is the case, stretching would not be advised initially as it could do more harm than good. Treatment and guidance may be essential from a practitioner who understands and can use the principles in this system.

12

Freedom

The results

I will never forget the look of wonder and amazement from Mrs Lewis, who had lower back and hip pain. She was so amazed at the benefits that she had after just one treatment.

> Mrs Lewis had been told many years earlier, after an X-ray of her hips, that her hip joints were severely degenerated. After suffering from pain and stiffness, she came for treatment to see if there was anything that could be done to help.
>
> She was amazed at the freedom of movement and elimination of pain achieved,

just by releasing some of the lower back and hip muscles. Literally, after one treatment of deep massage to the hip and spinal muscles, she felt so much freer and was pain-free.

The freedom that she experienced was not only physical but also in her attitude towards her body: she knew there was more she could do to help herself. She now has a complete programme of stretching that she can do to keep herself as free and active as possible.

Choosing the most appropriate health professional

You are responsible for your own body. Even with the best treatment in the world you will still need to do your part to care for yourself. However, some people want extra help from an appropriate and experienced health professional. This is a great way to get the best results, assuming you find someone who can work with this system.

If you are seeking help from a health professional it is critical that you find the right person – someone who understands the muscles' impact on your joints, and who has the specific knowledge to help you with this method.

In my opinion, the best practitioner to help you with this treatment is someone who uses and is familiar with Travell and Simons' myofascial trigger point manuals. If you struggle to find such a practitioner, the next best thing would be a practitioner skilled in muscle release techniques, such as a very good massage therapist or physical therapist who focuses mostly on muscle release. It is always a good idea to 'interview' the therapist first. Ask them how they work, to help ascertain if they are likely to be of significant benefit to your cause.

Usually we see results quicker when using a combination of effective muscle release through massage and trigger point release, rather than just muscle stretching on its own. Because of this I always recommend people use both treatments where possible.

The key is finding someone who understands what they are doing. You might ask a friend or family member to perform the massage, but to be more effective, I would suggest first asking an appropriate health practitioner to show them where and how to apply the massage. I would encourage you to have as much help from an appropriate health practitioner as possible, as the results are usually well worth the investment.

Where to from here?

My desire is that you will now use the information in this book to take action to help yourself and find the most freedom from your problem that is possible. Helping yourself may mean beginning a self-care programme with some stretch and self-massage at home.

If you choose to do this yourself, I reiterate: get the safety clearance from a medical practitioner first. This is to ascertain that your arteries or veins in the areas that you will be having stretched or massaged don't have clots or similar problems that could pose a health risk.

If you completed the review, record and restore chapters in this book, you should have a clearer idea of the level of severity of your OA, with some understanding of the muscle influence on this. You should have some knowledge about what can be done to help your muscles and subsequently your joints. You now have some very useful tools to help yourself.

However this book does not have the capacity to effectively show you all the muscles, stretches and massage techniques necessary for you to take care of your specific problem.

My aim is to make this method as accessible to as many people as possible. I believe the best way to do this is to keep the information as live as possible. To this end, I have compiled a complete comprehensive package, consisting of this book, a series of DVDs and accompanying workbooks. This information is the next best thing to having one-on-one consultation with me. It allows the information to be accessed by as many people as possible, almost anywhere in the world. To purchase the complete package, please visit www.freedomfromarthritis.com.

More help in your own home

The tools that I have compiled with DVDs and workbooks are fundamental in helping you help yourself even if you are receiving regular professional help.

If you don't have these resources from my complete self-treatment system, it is worth knowing that they can also be very useful even if you are being treated by a health practitioner, as you will understand more about your treatment and will be able to do a lot more to help yourself.

I have compiled these resources over 15 years and condensed them in to a very concise system specific for these problems. Other than those whom I train I don't know of anyone else in the world following these specific methods.

References and further reading

Alter, Michael J., *Sport Stretch*, 2nd edn, Human Kinetics, 1998

Barker, Vic, *Posture Makes Perfect*, Fitworld Publications, 1985

Bradley, Dinah and Dr Mike Thomas, *Hyperventilation Syndrome*, Kyle Books, 2011

Collins English Dictionary, New Zealand Edition, HarperCollins, 2011

Wilson, Dr James L. *Adrenal Fatigue: The 21st Century Stress Syndrome*. **Smart Publications, 2001**

Golomb, Beatrice, 'Statin adverse effects: A review of the literature and evidence for a mitochoncrial mechanism', *American*

Journal of Cardiovascular Drugs 2008:8(6): 373–418

Kendall, Florence Peterson, Elizabeth Kendall McCreary, Patricia Geise Provance, Mary McIntyre Rodgers and William Anthony Romani *Muscles: Testing and Function, with Posture and Pain*, Lippincott Williams and Wilkins, 2005

Statham, Bill, *The Chemical Maze, Shopping Companion: Your Guide to Food Additives and Cosmetic Ingredients*, 4th edn, Hyde Park Press, 2008

Simons, David G, Janet G Travell and Lois S Simons, *Travell and Simons' Myofascial Pain and Dysfunction: The Trigger Point Manual*, 2nd edn, 1999, Lippincott Williams and Wilkins

Murray, Michael, Joseph Pizzorno and Lara Pizzorno, *The Encyclopedia of Healing*

Foods, Piatkus Books, 2008

Soria, Cherie, Brenda Davis and Vesanto Melina, *The Raw Food Revolution Diet*, Healthy Living Publications, 2008